EyeRobics

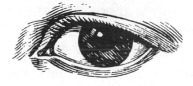

*How to improve
your vision*

MARILYN ROY

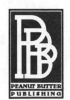

PEANUT BUTTER
PUBLISHING

Seattle, Washington
Portland, Oregon
Denver, Colorado
Vancouver, B.C.

Acknowledgements

The Author wishes to express appreciation to Dover Publications, Inc. for optical designs taken from *Optical and Geometrical Patterns and Designs* by Spyros Horemis.
5-D Stereogram created by Stephen Schutz, Ph.D. Published by Blue Mountain Arts, Inc., P.O. Box 4549, Boulder, Colorado 80306
Copyright © 1994 Stephen Schutz and Susan Polis Schutz. Reprinted with permission.

ISBN # 0-89716-712-0
Library of Congress 97-065740
A4.0047

Printed in the United States of America
10 9 8 7 6 5 4 3 2
First Printing April 1997
Second Printing February 1998

Peanut Butter Publishing
Pier 55, Suite 301 • 1101 Alaskan Hwy, Seattle, WA 98101
Old Post Office Bldg., 510 SW Third, Portland, OR 97201
Cherry Creek, 50 S. Steele, Suite 850, Denver, CO 80209
Ste. 230, 1333 Johnson Street, Pier 32, Granville Island, Vancouver BC V6H 3R9
e-mail: pnutpub@aol.com
Internet: http://www.pbpublishing.com

Table of Contents

Foreword
Dr. William L. Weis

I still remember sitting late at night in the old limestone library at Bowling Green, making sure that if I failed my freshman year in college it would not be for lack of effort. About the only time during my eighteen-hour days that my eyes weren't focusing on a book or writing tablet was in class, when I occasionally glanced up at my professors or at the overhead projection screen.

Halfway through my freshman year, my eyes started to protest. First, I had trouble focusing my two eyes together. This would happen every night about 9:00 P.M.—after ten to twelve hours of close work. The words in my books just wouldn't hold still unless I closed one or the other of my eyes. Then I noticed the people and the furnishings in the old library were losing their definition—my distance world was getting blurry and my close-up world wouldn't hold still!

My family had always believed in pursuing the "best" medical care available, so I made an appointment for an eye examination with a board-certified ophthalmologist (they were called oculists then). He examined my eyes and listened sympathetically to my sad story about losing my vision every night following a mere ten to twelve hours of uninterrupted close-up focusing. He nodded with a calmness and understanding that gave me assurance that the deterioration of my vision was perfectly normal and expected—after all, I was eighteen years old. It was time to enter the adult world of corrective lenses. There was not the slightest suggestion that my loss of visual acuity was even partially under my control. It obviously had nothing to do with the fact that I started abusing my eyes every day at 7:00 A.M. and didn't stop until my focus was so impaired—by 9:00 or 10:00 P.M.—that there was nothing left for me to do but go to bed.

I noticed that many of my friends were experiencing a similar "maturing" of their visual acuity—in fact, there was an epidemic of myopia sweeping through the university! We were all losing our abilities to see in the distance and it was, from all we could detect from talking with our eye doctors, a purely uncontrollable phenomenon. It just happens at a certain age (for many eighteen seemed to be the magic year) and we were just lucky we hadn't been afflicted sooner.

That was thirty years ago. What followed for me was a lifetime of gradually worsening myopia (near sightedness) as I continued to strain my eyes over long hours of close work and let progressively stronger lenses take care of my loss of distance vision. But at age forty-two, I made a fatal decision that would cause more deterioration in my vision over the next five years than had occurred over the previous twenty-two years since I first began wearing glasses.

My employer, Seattle University, added a "vision care" benefit to my compensation package. I hadn't had my eyes examined for a number of years, so I immediately looked in the yellow pages for a board-certified ophthalmologist I could walk to from our campus. His office was on the second floor of a small two-story building two blocks away. On the first floor was another business—an optical products dispensary.

I had my eyes examined and was pleased that I had

no apparent eye diseases—pleased, but not surprised, since serious eye diseases are relatively uncommon. However, in examining my vision, my doctor determined that my lens prescription should be strengthened. For convenience, I purchased my new glasses in the optical dispensary on the first floor. After all, my doctor's office was nice enough to offer me a "$20 off" coupon for glasses purchased downstairs.

I remember being impressed by two things from that visit. First, I was pleasantly surprised at how reasonable were the fees for my eye examination. I expected to pay at least twice the amount of the actual invoice. Second, I was unpleasantly surprised at how pricey glasses had become. It seemed like a lot of money for one pair of lenses and frames.

Now my story becomes unhappy. Within a matter of months, I began experiencing significant eye strain and further loss of my distance vision. I was so alarmed by the rapid deterioration that I went back to my doctor, even though my insurance for another examination required at least a year between visits. He checked my eyes and confirmed what I already knew: I needed even stronger lenses due to a rapid change in my myopia. He assured me that this was nothing to be alarmed about, that these periods of deterioration "often come in spurts" at about your age. I felt eighteen all over again—losing my eye sight through no fault of my own. I just happened to hit the magic age of forty-two and, presto, time for my DNA-programmed vision loss.

But it was just beginning. My eyestrain got worse. By evening, my eyes felt fatigued and overworked. And, often by noon, my eyes become so tired that I needed my strong distance lenses to see clearly only a few feet away. Fortunately, it didn't cost me very much to go back repeatedly to my ophthalmologist to be reassured that this loss of distance vision was perfectly normal in a man of my age. Sometimes I could buy this reassurance for a mere $30—a nice concession when my insurance wouldn't cover such frequent re-examinations.

As I saw it, there was only one "winner" in this dismal scenario: the optical dispensary on the first floor. I sort of felt sorry for my doctor. Truth was that for every dollar I spent upstairs getting my eyes examined, I spent $8 down below! (I keep careful records.) All the money in this eye care business was going to the glasses and contact lens makers and sellers—very little went to the hard-working certified ophthalmologists!

As fate would have it, in the midst of this phase of rapid vision loss, I talked with Marilyn Roy about her response to her own deteriorating vision. She had been wearing contact lenses for twenty years. When the last set she was using were too weak to correct her myopia, she decided to restore her natural eyesight rather than stay on the squirrel wheel of buying ever stronger contact lenses.

Of course, I thought she was crazy. "Don't you know," I argued, "that your eyes just naturally get weaker with age? There's nothing you can do about it." But she wasn't convinced. And after a year of practicing with the techniques she presents in this book, she called me to report that she had just passed her driver's test and could drive an automobile without corrective lenses! She was forty-five years old and had worn glasses and contact lenses for over twenty years!

I was astounded. In my thirty years of paying the extra bucks to consult with certified ophthalmologists, never had it been suggested to me that I had some responsibility for my vision fitness. No one ever suggested that I could consciously slow the deterioration of my vision, let alone that I could actually restore lost visual acuity.

Why? Why didn't my doctor tell me that eye strain—eye abuse in my case—contributed to my loss of acuity? Why hadn't anybody told me about people like Marilyn Roy, who take personal responsibility for their own visual fitness and do something about it?

I'm a business school professor, so often when I ask "Why?" my mind goes to business explanations. And to business questions. For example:

> 1. Where is the money in the "vision care" industry?

> Answer: In optical products, where profit margins are astronomical. Where contact lenses that cost pennies to make are sold for 100s of times their cost to produce. Also in surgery, where both the risks and the long-term benefits of treatment are problematical.

> 2. Is there any money in natural vision improvement?

> Answer: No. None.

> 3. Is there money in eye deterioration?

> Answer: Yes—in fact, that's where all the money is. During my own five years of rapid

vision loss, I spent over $1,000 on lenses, frames, and contact lenses—and only about $100 on eye examinations.

But there remained a lingering, troubling question. Why didn't my ophthalmologist tell me about vision therapy as a way of taking some responsibility for my own vision? I would gladly have paid him his modest fee either way. I would have gladly paid him more for such advice!

Then I started thinking bad thoughts—the kind we like to suppress. Not for one moment did I want to think that my gentlemanly licensed ophthalmologist might be taking referral kick-backs from downstairs! Professional medical ethics certainly wouldn't tolerate that. Right?

Well, I still don't know whether that's right or not. But as it turned out, my eye doctor was definitely not taking kickbacks from the optical dispensary downstairs. Of course, he didn't need to. He owned the optical dispensary!

My ophthalmologist is not unique in his dabbling at several levels in the "eye care" industry. Ownership in optical supplies dispensaries among certified ophthalmologists and optometrists is widespread and endemic to the "eye care" industry in America. Often, the cost of eye examinations is simply a loss-leader to get customers for the purchase of optical products and services: glasses, contact lenses, ever-changing frame styles, and corrective surgery. I wish I had known that five years ago. I now have a drawer full of prescription glasses that, thankfully, I have "outgrown" as a result of applying a mere fraction of the suggestions presented in this book. I now am driving my car with glasses that have prescription lenses that are a mere third of the strength before I started to take personal responsibility for my vision health. And I haven't even begun to do the exercises that Marilyn Roy recommends in this book—exercises that removed "corrective lenses" from her driver's license in one year!

By working with approximately five percent of the recommendations contained in this volume—those that take absolutely no time from my work day—I am now seeing better than I did "four prescriptions" ago, and my eyes now never feel strained or fatigued. Just over a year ago my evening activities were a visual blur. I had to wear strong lenses to function effectively in virtually every activity of my day. Now I am again teaching without glasses-and seeing my graduate students clearly. I am playing goalie for two soccer teams under the lights—and I can see the ball at both ends of the field! Today it wouldn't even occur to me to wear glasses playing basketball—two years ago I had no choice.

It all reduces to one simple analogy. I have responsibility for all aspects of my physical well being. Long ago I decided to take the time, regularly, to leave my office and my computer to go to our school gym for physical workouts. I could have chosen to stay in my office; the consequences would have been further muscle atrophy, higher body-fat density, higher blood pressure and resting heart beat, and a dismal fitness profile.

Two years ago, I decided to try reversing my rapidly deteriorating vision, following the advice of this book's author. Without that decision, I would today have a drawer of "outgrown" glasses for the opposite reason—because my eyes would have continued to worsen.

Put simply, it makes little sense to exercise care for all parts of my body except for my eyes. Vision is a gift—a wonderful gift. I know now that I have personal responsibility for and personal control over the care of that gift.

And so do you. This book will show you how to give yourself something very special—the gift of better vision. You can improve your vision. That is a fact. Unfortunately, you probably right now are doubting this assertion. And you doubt it because all the money in the eye care business is made by selling you "corrective" lenses and "corrective" surgery. So you have been told, indirectly or otherwise, that the only remedy for weak vision is to buy crutches—not to care for and exercise your eyes.

I suppose we can all be grateful that the money made each year from performing bone-setting surgery far exceeds the money made selling crutches and wheelchairs! Or else routine leg fractures would never be repaired and we would spend our remaining years using crutches and wheelchairs. Of course we would probably call them "corrective" devices instead of what they really are: crutches.

Yet that's what we are doing with our eyes. Abusing them until they become weak, and then accelerating the cycle of abuse and deterioration through ever-more-powerful "corrective" lenses. Stop the cycle. Reclaim responsibility for your own vision fitness. Consult your ophthalmologist for detention and treatment of eye diseases—thankfully very rare in our culture—but stop short of turning over personal responsibility for your eyesight to anyone who may be profiting from its continuing deterioration.

Part 1 — Self Assessment

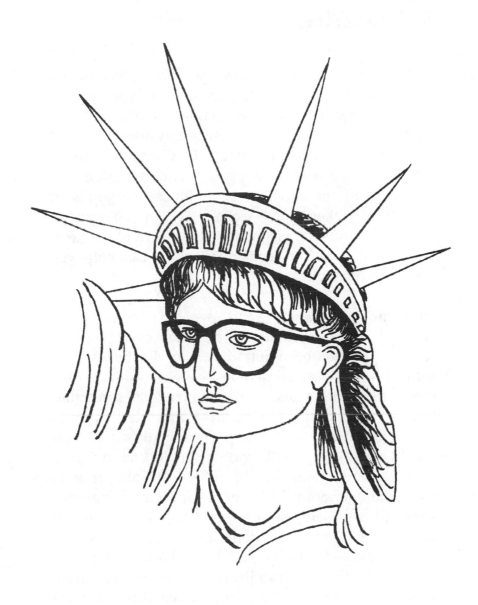

America Needs Better Vision

Introduction

Vision fitness is part of physical fitness, yet in our culture sixty percent of the population rely on glasses to see clearly. It is estimated that ninety percent of all individuals in the U.S. will eventually use glasses at some point in their lifetimes. In China the rising incidence of vision problems in children prompted educators to incorporate vision fitness programs in schools. Are there some techniques you can learn to maintain or regain vision fitness? Current research shows that there are techniques which can help you improve your sight.

Over the past twenty years, we have witnessed a physical fitness revolution which has overtaken our country. We've been introduced to the benefits of aerobic exercises, stretching, weight training, and yoga, along with a host of other recreational programs. Without exception we found these activities beneficial to our health and well being. Those individuals most caught up in this health craze stand in line at health fairs to have their hearts, lungs, fat and muscle measured and monitored. Doesn't it seem strange that after all this emphasis on fitness, we could so completely ignore the condition of our eyesight? Perhaps this is due to the outdated, but long held belief, that poor eyesight was an irreversible condition. I have written this book to help you prove that for most people vision fitness is as attainable a goal as is general body fitness.

What's Your Story?

There was probably a time you can remember before you needed to wear glasses. Seeing clearly was automatic and something you didn't think about very often. When did this end for you and what was happening in your life when you started wearing glasses?

If you cannot remember exactly, get out an old family photo album and start paging through it. You will probably come across many pictures that will help you recall what your life was like about that time. You may be able to pin point the exact year by looking at old school photos, or you may recall events of the time from vacation or holiday pictures. Now you might find your reaction, to your glasses quite different than your original reaction to wearing them when you were younger. Some people may notice that, in the early years, they did not consistantly wear glasses in all the photos around that time period. Maybe the glasses were not a permanent feature until much later. It might also be interesting to notice whether other family members or friends were wearing glasses at this time.

I feel that each of us has a story and it is important to recall this information, because understanding the problem may help you in your quest to become less dependent on glasses. It might also give you some information about habits and beliefs that you once had or have developed concerning your vision. You may find you'll recall many more details if you actually write down your story in a journal. This way you can add details later that may not seem significant now. You can use this journal later to track your progress, note significant insights and record your beliefs and frustrations while you are working to improve your sight.

I'll recount my story for you just to give you some idea of what I mean by recalling your history. I began wearing glasses in the fifth grade to see the blackboard from the back of the room. My first pair of glasses had light blue, metal frames. I liked them and wore them for everything. My sister and parents had been wearing glasses for some time before that. By the time I was in seventh and eighth grade, I see that I was not wearing glasses in school photos. By high school, I had stopped wearing glasses. I did not rely on them again until I was twenty-three. This time I got glasses to take the driving test and wore them infrequently outside of the car. In my early twenties, I started working as an accountant during the day and I was also attending night school. Now that I think about it, being myopic is a pretty good definition for an accountant. At that time, however, I had not yet come to realize this obvious correlation. For the next twenty years, I wore glasses or contacts and occasionally visited my eye doctor for a stronger prescription. The deterioration in my sight had been as high as 20/100 in my late thirties. I also had an astigmatism correction.

At the age of forty, I changed my work schedule from full-time to part-time. Also I had started studying art and was spending three to six hours a week drawing or painting from models, which required constant refocusing from far to near. These changes in my daily routine meant that I was spending less time doing close work and more time looking into the distance. When I turned forty-two, my eye doctor noted that my distance vision had improved slightly which was something I was glad to hear.

One day I just happened to come across a copy of *The Bates Method for Seeing Without Glasses*. I read parts of it and started experimenting with the ideas that very night. I had recently been having trouble with my contacts fogging up and I was looking for some alternative to wearing glasses for the rest of my life. Two weeks later, I left for a hiking trip in England. I didn't leave my glasses at home, but I vowed that I would try to get along without glasses during the trip as an experiment. I actually had no problems. Things were a little blurred but I didn't get lost.

When I first started working to restore my sight, I did not do many exercises other than not wearing my glasses, unless it was absolutely necessary, and checking my sight everyday with an eye chart. Instead of exercises, I tried to integrate seeing better into my daily life. If I was walking down the street, I would try to read all the signs or try to see people in the next block. If I was watching TV or a movie, I would focus on seeing peoples' eyes clearly or I would try reading the fine print on news shows. Within months, I started moving the TV farther away.

Within four months of going without glasses, I noticed that my eye muscles were letting me know when they were trying to see more. These strange little pulls or sensations around my eyes spurred me on because I knew my eyes were starting to adjust to seeing more at a distance. I was seeing more clearly and I continued to make progress until I decided to work another tax season. During this time, I found it difficult to keep my gains with the intense full-time close work. After tax season, I reverted again to only doing close work part-time. It took me exactly thirteen months in total until I was able to pass the driver's license vision test without lenses. This test requires 20/40 vision. In the last six months before passing the test, I started using Brian Severson's

Vision Freedom method in which you use plus glasses to add resistance while reading. It helps train your eyes to become more flexible and stronger. This method gave me the additional power to be able to pass the driver's test. I'm still working with astigmatism in one eye, but I'm also still noticing a natural improvement over time.

When I think about the story of how I lost my perfect sight, I realize that my eyes were working well all the time. When I was a full-time accountant, I was requiring them to do intense close work for long periods of time and they accommodated very well by becoming myopic. Once I started wanting to see far again, they adjusted to become more flexible in a short time.

It's not easy to get used to not wearing glasses if you have been relying on them for years and clear vision is not immediate, but the rewards of reclaiming your vision are well worth the time and effort.

Staying With It

The single most important element in any exercise program is maintaining motivation day after day for a long enough period so that the new behavior becomes a habit. Eventually small repetitions can lead to major improvements in fitness when integrated into your daily life. These are some of the ways I stayed motivated.

I found that practicing to see farther into the distance kept me from being bored while waiting in lines or doing routine tasks. I got my family and friends involved hoping their insights might help me improve my techniques. I continued to find that others were instinctively intrigued with the concepts and immediately wanted to tell me about how they lost their perfect sight. I frequently find visitors spontaneously checking their own vision with the charts I have posted in the hall. Children never fail to turn this into a game.

It took me no time at all to convince my husband that he might also be able to become less dependent on glasses. He tried several of the things I suggested and has reverted to wearing an old, much weaker, prescription. He also finds that his eyes feel much less stressed by the end of the day.

In my quest to keep motivation high, I decided to teach a class in these techniques in the local evening community education program. I've had a great response to my class. Over sixty students have attended and there continues to be a lot of interest in the course. I began developing this book as a learning tool for the class. Since I have now incorporated all the course material into this manual, it can be used as an independent self-help course at home.

Getting Started

The first step in designing a program that will benefit you is to determine your current ability to perform some simple vision tests. Don't become disillusioned if you cannot see the chart from the prescribed distance without your glasses. Just adjust your distance until you can read some of the letters and record the approximate distance you are from the chart. If you have mounted the chart on the wall, you might want to place a piece of tape on the floor marking this point. This will be your baseline measurement from which you will measure your progress. Attempt to do each test and record your results. Be sure to keep and date this written record of your results for comparison later, because nothing will keep you motivated more than seeing measurable progress toward your goals.

The self-test begins on the next page. You can do the test both with your glasses on and off so that you can note the differences in the way you see with and without your glasses.

When I first tested myself, I was surprised to see that I had trouble seeing the 20/20 line even with my glasses on. As I progressed, I found it interesting to notice the greater clarity that I had achieved both with and without my glasses. Soon I was able to see the 20/15 line clearly with my glasses on.

Measuring distance vision or acuity is usually the first test most people think of when they have their eyesight checked, but this is only one measurement that is important in seeing clearly. In the test, I also include questions on clarity, reading acuity, eye dominance, and the ability to process images with both eyes.

Please turn to the next page and complete the self-test before reading further. It is important to determine specifically what your needs are before proceeding, so that you will be able to decide what information and exercises are relevant to you. For example, problems relating to astigmatism probably will have little relevance to those who are farsighted, since astigmatisms, which need corrective lenses, are almost always in nearsighted individuals.

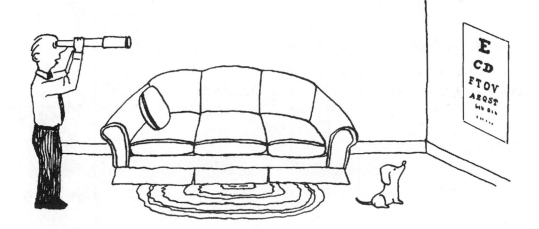

Vision Self Test - Baseline Chart

Use this chart to record answers to the test questions which begin on the following page.

Date	Without Glasses			With Glasses	
	Both eyes	Right eye	Left eye	Right eye	Left eye

1. Distance Acuity

2. Clarity:
a. Shadows or Double Vision?
b. Blurred - no sharp edges?
c. Sensitivity to bright light?

3. Reading Acuity

4. Astigmatism Test
a. Horizontal Lines Clearer?
b. Vertical Lines Clearer?

5. Processing Images

6. Eye Dominance

Vision Self Test

Record your answers on the Baseline Chart located on the previous page.

1. Distance Acuity

Use the Wall Chart on page 15 to determine the smallest line of print that you can see standing twelve feet from the chart.

2. Clarity

A. Do you see any double images or shadows of other letters in the white spaces?

B. Do the edges of the letters appear to be crisp and clear or are the edges grey and blurred?

C. Are you sensitive to bright lights? Do you need to wear sunglasses often?

3. Reading Acuity

Find the reading chart which is located on page 17. Hold the reading chart approximately fourteen inches from your eyes and determine the smallest row of characters that you can read. You should be able to read the smallest line if you have perfect reading vision.

4. Astigmatism Test: Distance Distortion of Horizontal, Verticle, or Diagonal Lines

Use the geometric designs on the bottom part of the reading chart to see the effects of astigmatism. Hold the designs at reading distance or move them farther away. If you have astigmatism you will notice shadows, blurs, or distortions through parts of the design while other parts will appear clearer. (You may need to place the designs on the floor and view them from a standing position to see the distance effect.)

(The test is continued on the next page.)

Vision Self Test (continued)

5. Processing Images with Both Eyes

Look at an object such as a chair or lamp ten to twenty feet from you. Now bring your finger up in front of your face while you are still focusing on the object. Notice in the foreground you see two fingers. Now focus on your finger and notice in the background there are now two chairs (this is what you are doing when you cross your eyes.) If you do not see the two chairs or two fingers when you do this exercise, your brain may not be processing the messages from both of your eyes.

6. Eye Dominance

Use a pencil to punch a hole in a piece of paper. Now look at an object across the room. Bring the paper with the punched hole in front of your eyes so that you can see the object through the hole. Close one eye. If you can still see the object, the open eye is your dominant eye. If you cannot see the object your other eye is your dominant eye.

Wall Chart

C E	20/100
F B T	20/70
E D K A	20/50
R O P N S X	20/40
T U Y G Z D R	20/30
F L S E Q A C P	20/25
B O T N G Z H F	20/20
S N R G V O P F L	20/15
P E T F D O C L	20/10

Mount this chart on a wall where there is an artificial light source and the
lighting is consistent day and night. Stand 12 feet from the chart to test vision.

This page was intentionally left blank so that you can remove the eye chart and mount it on the wall.

Reading Chart

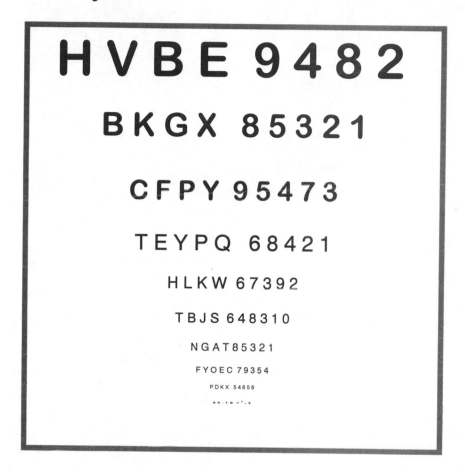

HVBE 9482

BKGX 85321

CFPY 95473

TEYPQ 68421

HLKW 67392

TBJS 648310

NGAT85321

FYOEC 79354

PDKX 54658

++·+ ⁼ ⁻`·+

Geometric Designs

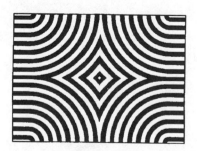 

Reading Chart

HVBE 9482

BKGX 85321

CFPY 95473

TEYPQ 68421

HLKW 67392

TBJS 648310

NGAT85321

FYOEC 79354

PDKX 54658

Geometric Designs

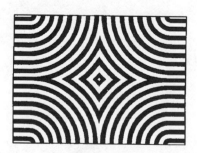
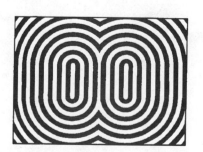

Part II — Mechanics and Theory

Basic Structure of the Eye

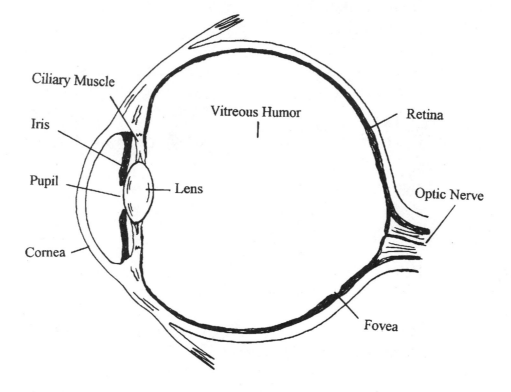

Ciliary Muscle

Iris

Pupil

Cornea

Vitreous Humor

Lens

Retina

Optic Nerve

Fovea

How Eyes Work

Refer to the diagram of the eye on the prior page as you read through this description of the basic structure of the eye. The **cornea** is the clear covering on the outside of the eye. It serves as a protective shield, but it has another important function. Because it is round in shape, it also serves as a lens which does most of the focusing of the light rays as they enter the eye. The **iris**, which is the colored part of the eye, is a muscle that regulates the amount of light entering the eye. The iris expands and contracts the size of the pupil allowing more light to enter the pupil in dim conditions, but reducing the size of the pupil to allow less light into the eye in bright conditions. The black **pupil** is an aperture, or opening in the eye, through which light enters. Behind the pupil, the light passes through a **lens** which changes shape to focus the image on the retina. The **ciliary muscle**, which is an involuntary muscle, forms a circular ban around the lens. It contracts to pull the lens into a convex shape while reading or looking close and relaxes to allow the lens to take on a flatter or even concave shape to focus in the distance. Before the light rays hit the retina, they pass through the **vitreous humor,** which is a clear gelatinous material filling the interior of the eyeball. Finally, light reaches the **retina,** which is a multilayered light-sensitive membrane lining the inner eyeball. It transmits the information through the **optic nerve** to the brain where the image is translated so that we recognize what we are seeing. When the image is focused on the **fovea**, a particularly sensitive area of the retina, a very distinct image will be seen.

Diagram of the Exterior Muscles of the Eye

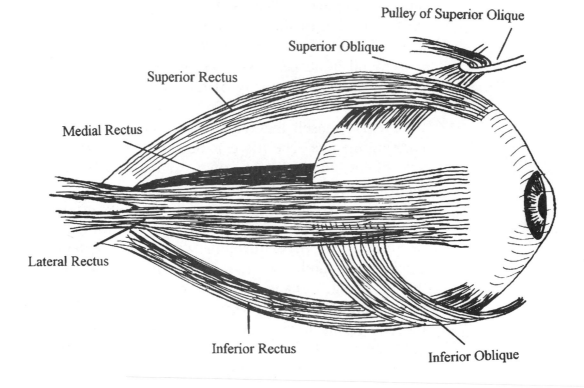

Pulley of Superior Olique

Superior Oblique

Superior Rectus

Medial Rectus

Lateral Rectus

Inferior Rectus

Inferior Oblique

Exterior Muscles of the Eye

There are six, large, voluntary muscles on the outside of the eyeball. The four recti muscles attach to the outer layer of the eyeball. They are approximately evenly spaced around the eye and pull directly over the top, bottom and sides of the eyeball. The two oblique muscles form an almost complete band around the middle of the eyeball. In relation to the size of other muscles in the body, these six muscles have been described as being 100 times as powerful as necessary to do the tasks they are expected to perform.

These muscles are responsible for changing the shape of the eye, which is necessary to change the focus from near to far. They also allow us to change the direction of our gaze. As seen in the muscles in the rest of our body, the recti and oblique muscles work as opposing forces. The oblique muscles wrap around the eyeball and when contracted they elongate the eye to see close. The recti muscles pull back on the cornea when contracted to flatten or shorten the eye to see far. The eye shortens to see far and elongates to see close just like one adjusts a pair of binoculars. The oblique muscles are involved in producing nearsightedness. The recti are involved in producing astigmatism and farsightedness.

Common Refractive Errors

Refractive errors occur when something causes the light rays to focus on a point other than the retina. When this happens the person sees a blurred or distorted image rather than a clear and focused image. Refractive errors usually are caused by tense muscles that keep the eye from relaxing enough to automatically refocus from near to far or visa versa. Over time these tensed muscles can actually reshape the cornea and eyeball so that they no longer return to a perfectly round shape, while the opposing muscles lose coordination or became weak so they no longer correct the problem. A person with refractive errors has really only lost muscle coordination and flexibility. Even if the shape of the eye has changed, the condition is reversible. Following is a description of the most common refractive errors.

Normal Sight
Focus point is on the retina.

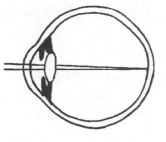

Farsighted (Hyperopia)
Focus point is beyond the retina. The eyeball is slightly short.

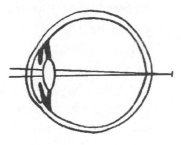

Nearsighted (Myopia)
Focus point is short of the retina. The eyeball is elongated.

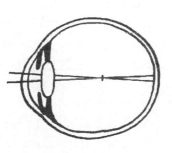

Astigmatism
There are multiple focal planes due to an irregularly shaped cornea. If a correction is needed for astigmatism, the person is usually nearsighted.

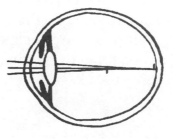

Nearsightedness: (or Myopia)

A nearsighted person can see to read and do close work, but has trouble seeing the eye chart twenty feet away. When a nearsighted person focuses to read he has no problem, his eye elongates so that the image falls directly on the retina. When he tries to see far, his eye remains too elongated causing the light rays to come into focus at a point in front of the retina. The image is blurred because the light rays begin again to diverge behind the focus point. The physical cause of the blur may be due to several things. The oblique muscle, which if not relaxed, could hold the eyeball in an elongated position. Pressure in the eye, from not relaxing, may have caused the cornea to become too steeply curved or the ciliary muscles may not be able to relax enough to allow the lens to flatten. Many studies have been done which have shown a high correlation between myopia and doing a lot of reading or other close work. If the eye muscles do not relax completely for far focus, the eye is held in this contracted state, and the person is over focusing for distance. Dr. Joseph Trachtman, inventor of a devise to cure myopia, has shown that merely being able to relax the ciliary muscle can improve nearsightedness significantly. Eighty per cent of people wearing glasses are nearsighted and most develop this condition by the time they are in their early twenties.

Farsightedness: (or Hyperopia)

This person can see far but has trouble focusing to read. In farsightedness, the person has no problem seeing the eye chart because the eye shortens enough to see into the distance, but when he tries to read, the eye does not lengthen enough causing the light rays to come into focus at a point behind the retina so the image appears blurred. The physical cause of the blur may be due to the recti muscles not being able to relax enough which causes the eyeball to be too short or the cornea to be too flat. Another problem may be that the ciliary muscle may not be able to contract enough to bend the lens to clearly focus. The nearsighted eyeball is definitely elongated, but the farsighted eyeball is only slightly shorter than normal. In farsightedness, the person is under focusing for close work.

Near Far Vision:

Some people have one eye which is able to see far and one eye which is adapted to seeing close. This is called near far vision.

Presbyopia: (literally Old Person's Sight)

This condition is the gradual loss of accommodative power for close work. Somewhere between the ages of forty to fifty, it is common to experience trouble focusing to read. Most authorities attribute this to the lens becoming less flexible as we age. Consequently the ciliary muscles begin to have difficulty bending the lens to focus close. Even those who are nearsighted are affected by presbyopia.

Astigmatism

If you think you have an especially peculiar case because you have an astigmatism correction, don't let that fact disturb you any longer. Actually, astigmatism is the most common refractive error and it occurs in ninety percent of all eyes. Astigmatisms that need correction, however, are typically associated with myopia. No eye is perfectly round, but an eye that has perfect vision has a smooth round cornea which focuses the light rays together just as a magnifying glass focuses a beam of sunlight. Astigmatism is created because the recti muscles are pulling unevenly causing the cornea to become more elliptically shaped. Usually, the cornea has taken on a steeper curve or arch across the diameter either along the horizontal or vertical axis. This irregular curvature causes some light rays to focus in front of the retina while others may focus farther back. The image appears distorted due to the multiple focal planes. The blur zones caused by astigmatisms can be seen when one views a geometric design. You may see the parallel curving lines clearly on some parts of the design, but blur zones may distort other parts of the image. If the cornea is round, all the lines will appear equally clear. If the cornea is unevenly curved, horizontal lines may fade out, vertical lines may fade out, or diagonal lines may fade out. Astigmatisms can be diminished by relaxing the eye.

Distortions due to Astigmatism

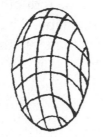

More steeply curved left to right

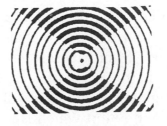

At a distance vertical lines blur

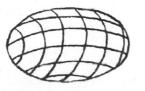

More steeply curved top to bottom

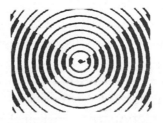

At a distance horizontal lines blur

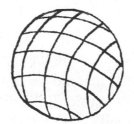

Evenly rounded

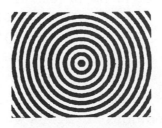

At a distance all lines equally clear

How to Read Prescriptions

Lens powers are measured in diopters. The higher the number, the stronger the lens. Pluses are used to indicate reading glasses or magnifying lenses. Minuses are used for indicating distance or reducing lenses. Magnifying lenses are convex in shape. They bow out and are thicker in the middle than on the edges. Minus lenses are concave and bow in so they are narrower in the center than at the edges. For astigmatism, the lens will have an additional cylinder ground into it which is aligned to compensate for the opposite cylindrical formation of the eye.

A prescription might be written like this:
O.D. (right eye) -2.25 -.50 x 175 degrees
O.S. (left eye)　 -2.00 -.25 x 175 degrees
add O.U. (each eye) +1.50

This prescription is for bifocals. The right eye needs a nearsighted correction of -2.25, and an astigmatism correction of -.50 at 175 degrees. The left lens is slightly weaker, only needing a -2.00 nearsighted correction and a -.25 astigmatism correction. In addition, a magnification correction of +1.50 is made on each lens for reading.

Roughly speaking 20/100 vision needs -1.00 correction, 20/200 a -2.00 correction; however, prescriptions may be stronger to insure that the patient has perfect vision in the worst possible lighting conditions. Eyeglasses do not actually correct the images that your eye sees, they create distortions in proportion. Concave lenses reduce the size of the images you see and convex lenses magnify the images. Cylinders produce some distortion even though they are aligned to compensate for the irregular shape of the eye.

Corrective Lenses

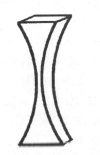

Nearsighted Correction
Concave Lens

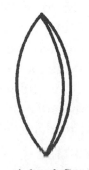

Farsighted Correction
Convex Lens

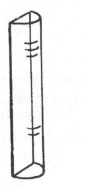

Astigmatism Correction
Cylindrical Lens

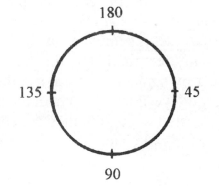

Angle of astigmatism is
measured on a 180 degree circle

The Eye Chart

Herman Snellen, a Dutch ophthalmologist, designed the first eye chart in the 1860s. The only objective of the chart is to determine how much distance acuity we have. Although our eyes were designed for distance vision, we now rarely use our eyes to see that small of detail at a distance of twenty feet. The 20/20 line was established to demonstrate the size of print a person, with good eyesight, could read standing twenty feet away. Twenty feet was used because light rays entering the eye at that distance are parallel, and our eyes are not required to bend the rays to focus them on the retina. The eye would function the same way for light rays past twenty feet so it is not necessary to test our sight at a farther distance. If someone has 20/100 sight, the smallest line he can read, could be seen at 100 feet by someone with good eyesight. Likewise, if someone has 20/15 vision, he can read at twenty feet the letters that can only be seen at fifteen feet by someone who meets the standard measure of good eyesight. If someone's eyesight can only be corrected to 20/200, they are considered legally blind. Only 20/40 vision is required to pass the driver's test.

How Pinhole Glasses Work

If you have trouble seeing without your glasses, you may find it amazing that you can see much better if you simply look through a pinhole punched in a piece of paper. The pinhole actually is focusing the light rays so they enter your eye as parallel lines, and your eye is not required to do as much focusing to see more clearly. This is the same concept that is used in pinhole glasses. Although they don't correct your vision, they will give you the experience of being able to see better without actually relying on corrective lenses.

Eye-Hand Dominance

Use the Vision Self Test to determine which is your dominant eye. The dominant eye has been shown to process information slightly faster than the non-dominant eye. Usually if you are right-eyed, you are also right-handed and visa versa, but some people have crossed dominance. This is common in baseball batters. You may find it interesting to concentrate on improving your eyesight as an extension of practicing your favorite sports activity. Better use of the eyes has been proven to improve an athlete's scoring ability. Probably the number one rule in sports is to keep your eye on the ball all the way through the play. You will find that different vision skills are used for different sports. For example reaction time is important in baseball, but not golf; peripheral vision is not important in archery.

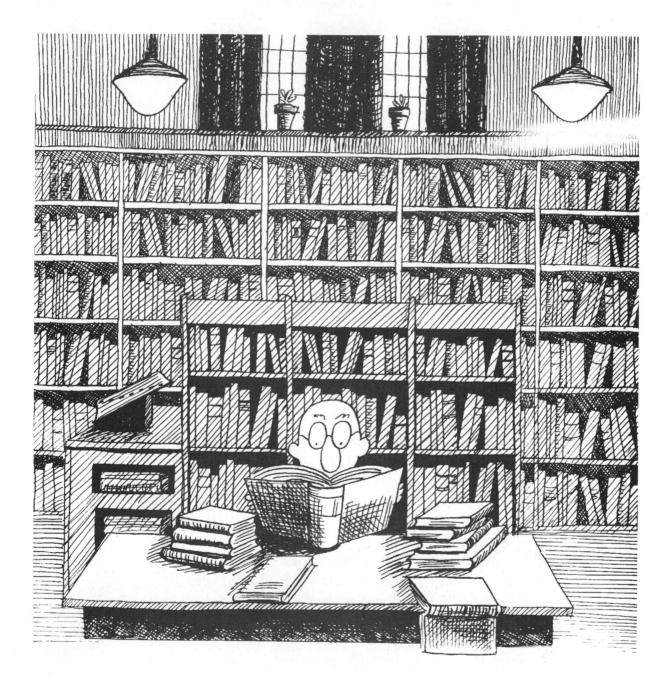

Historical Perspective

Myopia has been the primary vision problem afflicting young people since the early 1800s and continues to be the most common reason people need glasses. According to Doctors Seiderman and Marcus, in their book *20/20 Is Not Enough*, an ophthalmologist named James Ware had noted a high correlation between doing close work, such as reading, and nearsightedness as early as 1813. He was observing applicants for military service and found that twenty-five percent of Oxford students were nearsighted. (Now eighty percent of graduate students are nearsighted.)[1] The incidence of nearsightedness was far less frequent among the rest of the population, which included many farmers and fishermen. Since then, many other researchers have reported similar results from studies done on various cultures around the world. The statistics bear out the fact that although genetics may play a role, myopia is highly correlated with educational level, which requires intense close work.

Around the turn of the century a prominent American ophthalmologist, Dr. William Bates, developed a revolutionary model for explaining and treating vision problems. He proposed that vision problems were not caused by the mechanical factors within the eye but instead by a combination of physical, emotional and mental responses to our environment—basically the stress of modern civilization. He also noted the increase in vision problems as children went through the educational process. After studying thousands of patients with vision problems, Bates realized that

[1] T. Grosvenor, "The Results of Myopia Control Studies Have Not Been Encouraging," published in volume 4, no. 1 of the *Journal of Behavioral Optometry,* pages 17-19.

prescribing glasses was not a satisfactory solution to poor vision. Bates thought that when glasses were prescribed, the patient could immediately see better, but usually returned within a couple years only to require a higher prescription and the real problem of poor vision was not being addressed. Quoting from Bates, as written in Dr. Marilyn B. Rosanes-Berrett's book *Do You Really Need Glasses?*, "Myopia and hyperopia are not permanent, irremediable disabilities determined by the fixed shape of the eyeballs. Their shape is not fixed, it can change constantly in response to many factors, among them tense muscles. If an eyeball does not change its shape, it is because those muscles are tense from strain, and hold it rigid, or are flaccid from disuse or misuse, and exert no effect." In order to cure vision problems, Bates prescribed relaxation techniques, use of eye charts, and the mimicking of normal constant movement of healthy eyes, which includes blinking often.

Unfortunately, the Bates method was not accepted by the medical community in the early 1900s. Despite this setback, Bates' technique continued to be practiced and his book, *The Bates Method for Better Eyesight Without Glasses*, is still available in bookstores today. Aldous Huxley, author of *Brave New World*, wrote *The Art of Seeing* after successfully using the Bates method to overcome a near-blind condition. The techniques described in both books seem right in line with the recently popular holistic approach to healing. Since the 1940s, others have built on this research and methodology. Current books include many written by optometrists, educators and other lay people who have successfully cured themselves using similar techniques. These methods are being used in other countries also. The Bates Method is being taught primarily in England and India. However, other natural vision improvement practitioners can be found in Canada, Australia,

Germany, Belgium, Switzerland, the Netherlands, and Italy. Dr. Liberman noted in his recent book *Take Off Your Glasses and See*, in 1949, the Chinese government decided to do something to offset the rising incidence of myopia and initiated a program in schools and factories that devotes twenty minutes a day to eye exercises. The Chinese claim that this has reversed the increase in myopia in China.

For further study, see the bibliography in the back of the book for a list of other current books available in libraries and bookstores.

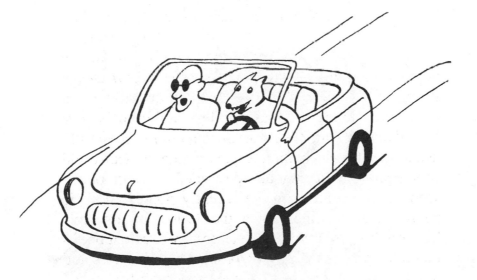

You're either steering your own course
or just along for the ride.

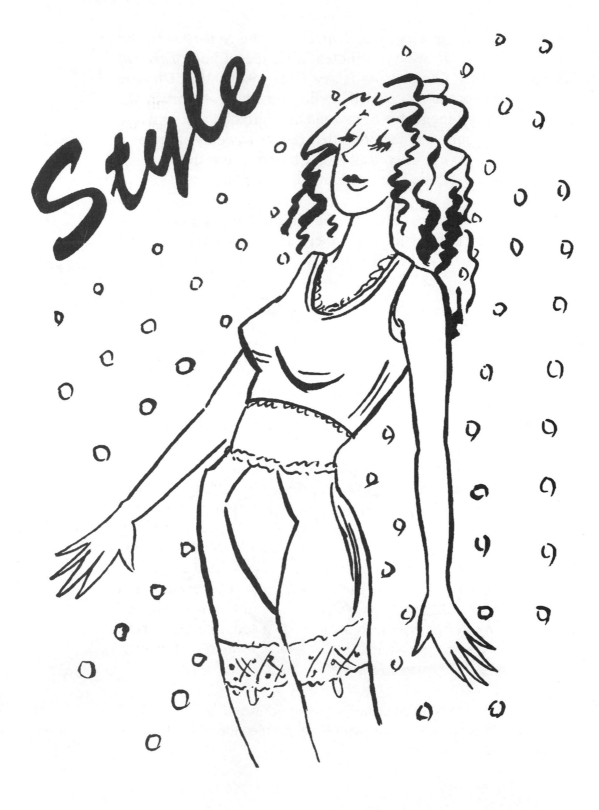

Consumer Beware

Before the craze of aerobics and ten minute abdominal videos, women relied on the fashion industry's solution for abdominal bulges. Remember the old advertisements for girdles in the 1950s which convinced women that the solution to a bulging stomach could be purchased in the lingerie section of any department store? Thanks to Jane Fonda and a number of other fitness instructors, women of the 1990s are no longer as gullible as they once were and realize that the only true solution for the lack of body fitness is an optimal exercise routine and lifestyle changes that support health and fitness.

Besides the obvious improvements exercise makes to our appearance, aficionados become addicted to the other rewards that come with it, including: better health, increased strength, more energy and an overall feeling of well being. In the longest running study of exercise and aging, Dr. Fred Kasch at San Diego State College has documented the fitness level of thirty men over twenty-three years comparing those who continue to exercise to those who stopped exercising. "Over twenty-three years, the regular exercisers lost fitness at one-third the annual rate of those who did not exercise," according to M. Elaine Cress, Ph.D. and research assistant professor of the University of Washington's Department of Medicine/Geriatrics. This was published in an article printed in the July, 1996 edition of *Northwest Prime Time Journal.*

Unfortunately, the eye products industry is no more ethical than any other big business in our free enterprise system. Selling more merchandise has become the goal in our consumer society. According to Richard Leviton in his book *Seven Steps to Better Vision*, "In 1990 Americans spent over $15 billion on eye care and prescription lenses." Eye care products have also fallen into the fashion marketing schemes. Often the eye exam is the least expensive part of a trip to the eye clinic. Prescriptions remain obscure and prevention and non-surgical correction of common refractive problems is never mentioned. (Until recent Washington State legislation in 1996, eye care specialists were not required to give patients a written copy of their prescriptions making it difficult for price comparison shopping.)

Now the optimum solution is the purchase of various optical devises or expensive surgery that offers an instant and effortless fix for the patient and a high monetary reward for the eye industry. But like the girdle, these solutions do nothing to address the prevention or reversal of poor sight. For many individuals, lack of any preventative action has actually resulted in a serious dependency on using glasses.

Ethical questions arise as to whether responsibility lies with eye care specialists to advise us on better eye fitness or is it an individual's responsibility to demand solutions that address the underlying problems rather than demanding an instant and effortless fix. Unfortunately, when there is a conflict of interest in the industry, as there is with some eye care specialists who run their own optical dispensaries, the incentive is to sell the product rather than offer advice on prevention or improvement.

Make Clearer Eyesight A Concious Daily Activity

We often take for granted the correct posture of a dancer during a performance, but movement instructors know that this is no accident. Correct body alignment is constantly and consciously practiced. All athletes learn that perfect body form, well balanced muscles, and effortless coordination will make the difference between being a winner or loser in competition. They take advantage of sophisticated computerized measurement systems to analyze their performances. You can use this same strategy in correcting your eyesight. It pays to become more discerning and aware of your own sight distortions.

Vision acuity usually declines at a gradual enough rate that, unless you pay close attention or measure it, you seldom are aware of the change until it interferes with your daily activities. If you wear the same glasses constantly you will probably find that you don't know much about the natural capabilities of your eyes. How far away can you recognize someone? Can you thread a needle without your glasses on? What special distortions do you create? Is it just blurry or do you see additional lines that aren't there?

Muscles of the body are remarkably adaptable, but they maintain only the amount of mass and strength you need to meet daily physical demands. Fortunately, for most people, good sight requires nothing more than maintaining the muscle balance and coordination with which we were born. Daily habits of how we use our eyes may make unclear sight due to irregular muscle form seem permanent but, because muscles are adaptable, when we begin changing our activities, our muscles will change, too. Be sure you consciously challenge those old habits and exercise your eyes every day, to see something, which is slightly out of focus, just a little clearer.

Computers & Eyestrain

I must admit to really liking computers. I was an early convert, purchasing one of the first Kaypro models of the personal computer in the early 1980s and, albeit with some struggling, I've tried to stay current. There is no doubt about it, personal computers have made my work much faster and more efficient. I'd never be able to move back to a manual typewriter or adding machine. But even though I enjoy computers, I still seem to notice some niggling little resistance to increasing the time I have to spend on them. Although it makes a lot of sense to eventually convert more and more printed material into computer files, I would hate to give up reading a printed copy of the morning newspaper. I also would have a hard time giving up the pleasurable experience of snuggling up on the couch with a good book or magazine. Sometimes I wonder if this is just my own knee-jerk reaction to moving into the high-tech age, but I think that the truth is that it is just not as relaxing working on the computer as it is reading a printed page. This is especially apparent when I am ready to do a final read through edit on the computer—I give up and print out a copy which I can read in a more comfortable and leisurely setting.

Generally speaking, optomitrists have reported that workers who use video display terminals have more visual focusing complaints than those viewing printed material and the complaints increase as the workers spend more hours at the computer. What are the most common problems people complain about? E.G. Goodwin and J.S. Hacunda have documented a list of both direct and indirect symptoms of VDT (video display terminal) induced visual stress in their book *Computers & Visual Stress*, 1990, including:

Eyestrain
Blurred Vision
Irritated Eyes
Headaches
Eye Focusing Problems
Double Vision
Color Perception Changes
Discomfort with Prescription Glasses
Nearsightedness

The indirect symptoms include:

Back, Neck, Shoulder or Arm Pain
Irritability
Increased Nervousness
Lowered Visual Efficiency

Do any of these problems reflect your own experiences? I've definitely noticed some of these symptoms.

Computer use is very demanding on our visual abilities. G. Murch used laser technology to study visual fatigue in computer users over time. He found that the eye cannot focus on the video terminal with the same accuracy as the printed page. Over a period of hours the computer user's focus point relaxed and extended beyond the screen causing the screen to appear less clear and harder to read. His findings were published in an article entitled "How Visible is Your Display?" in *Electo-Optical Systems Design*, 14 (3), 1982. It appears from the study that the computer image does not provide enough stimulus to cause the eye to accommodate effectively. In addition, clinical optometrists have found that a few computer users overfocus, which means they are focusing at a point in front of the screen so the image they see is not clear. Other computer users experience a breakdown of eye coordination skills which cause them to see double images after working on the computer for long periods. If an individual lacks the visual skill to see the image easily on a VDT screen, he may begin to tense his body and move his head in an attempt to focus in better. This may lead to posture related pains in the neck, shoulders or back. Because workers are not aware of ways to reduce VDT visual stress, they may begin to experience job burn out, high absenteeism or visual maladaptions such as nearsightedness or eyestrain.

Why do VDTs cause eyestrain?

1. When using a computer you are refocusing often between the key board, the screen and the copy. This requires more work for the eye muscles than just focusing on a book.

2. Older computer monitors have a slow fading phosphor glow which produces some flicker. The flickering image, when it is perceptible, is less restful to look at than a printed copy.

3. Often the monitor is not well positioned. The resting position for our eyes is a slightly downward angle. While reading or doing other close work, we usually naturally look down. Sometimes computer monitors are set up to be viewed looking straight ahead, which requires our eye to be less relaxed. The screen may also be quite close to our eyes. Optimally the computer screen should be positioned up to twenty-five inches away, which is further than one would hold a book.

4. Executives report less eyestrain than data entry workers or air traffic controllers who are required to intensely focus on the computer screen for long periods. Executives usually have more varied tasks and have more opportunity to refocus their eyes at a more restful distance.

5. Computer screens may reflect glare of other light sources which can make the screen harder to see.

6. Laptop computers are popular because of their portability, but the normal screen image is much reduced to fit on the small screen. Needing to focus on the smaller images is not as relaxing.

7. People using bifocals may have to raise or tilt their head to read the computer screen if their reading lens is positioned low on their glasses. This may cause neck or back pain.

8. Some type fonts are poorly defined on a computer screen because they have low dot matrix dimensions. This makes them harder to read.

9. Often, people forget to blink when they are concentrating on close work. For contact lens wearers, lack of blinking can cause their eyes to become dry. Controlled humidity in office buildings or computer areas may also contribute to this problem.

10. Using a computer may become more difficult for nearsighted contact wearers when they reach forty to fifty years of age. This is because their internal lens stiffens and makes it more difficult to focus close. Nearsighted contact wearers need to converge their eyes more and focus more than they do when they wear glasses because the contacts sit on the cornea rather than a half inch away.

11. It is unlikely that there is any radiation hazard from computers since UV and infrared radiation in sunlight are much greater than the levels present in front of a computer monitor.

12. If you have trouble crossing your eyes, you may have difficulty focusing on a computer monitor because you need to converge your eyes to see close clearly. Exercises crossing your eyes can improve your ability.

You can strengthen your eyes and improve your visual abilities for optimal computer use by doing the exercises in the last part of the book.

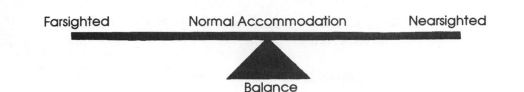

Farsighted   Normal Accommodation   Nearsighted

Balance

Maintaining Balance

Seeing clearly is part of balancing close work with more relaxed far focusing. As our work life continues to rely more on computers, the proliferation of information forces us to learn new ways to deal with large amounts of data. Most people experience some amount of visual fatigue doing close up tasks since our eyes were designed for distance vision in natural light. Optometrists call this strain near-point stress. Just maintaining balance in activities can play an important role in giving you plenty of visual variety and reducing near-point stress. Locating your desk or computer near a window might help remind you to look up and refocus often. Also the natural light, or as an alternative full spectrum lighting, appears to play a part in good visual acuity. Another way to increase visual variety is to balance close work with participation in sports or spectator events. Almost all sports give us the opportunity to track the players, follow the ball, and change focus often. Participation is the best alternative since it allows you to improve your overall body fitness rather than just the fitness of your eyes. It also gives you practice in visual-motor coordination.

Part III — Your Exercise Program

The Basics

1. As Bates proved, the eye is not fixed but is always changing shape to accommodate from near to far vision. The eye which has perfect sight is relaxed when it is focused for far and near vision. If you do not have clear sight, your eyes may be straining whether you are wearing glasses or not.

2. The brain works in conjunction with the eye giving feedback, which helps the eye bring things into clear focus.

3. Glasses mask the sight problem. The glasses make things *appear* clear, so the eye no longer needs to accommodate to the degree that it once did to focus clearly. Coordination and flexibility of the eye muscles may decline if the muscles are no longer required to work as hard to see clearly.

4. The exercises are to help the eye gain coordination and become more flexible again. There are relaxation exercises and accommodation (adjusting from near to far) exercises.

5. In order to regain vision fitness, you need to relearn to see without glasses. However, it is not usually possible to totally function without lenses if you have been relying on them for years and need them to drive or work safely. Start by using them only when you need them. Work towards relaxed seeing and being able to function at some tasks without glasses so that you begin to rely less on your glasses. You can use your old pair of glasses, with a weaker correction, as an interim step.

6. Develop an active interest in seeing clearly and you will begin to notice that even glasses distort things to some degree.

7. Balancing your day between using near and far vision is important. To remain flexible, the eye needs exercise in both areas.

8. Remember to give your eyes breaks from constant close work.

9. Blinking helps the eye change focus and lubricates the eye. Blinking and continually changing focus helps the eye relax. Staring puts a strain on the eyes. Try to develop the same movements of healthy eyes, blinking and changing focus often.

10. Don't wear distance glasses while reading. Wear reading glasses only for close work. When you read through distance glasses, your eyes must elongate an additional amount to accommodate for the strength of the prescription. When you focus far in reading glasses, your eyes must shorten an additional amount to accommodate for the lenses.

11. Get out of the habit of wearing sunglasses unless you are in a particularly bright glare, such as you find from snow or water. Sunglasses will make your eyes more sensitive to light. Foregoing sunglasses will help your eyes gain flexibility adapting to bright days.

12. Use the eye chart every day, preferably in the morning, to establish a baseline and monitor progress or regression. No matter how long you have worn glasses or how strong your prescription, you can improve your vision.

Designing a Training Program

1. Devise your exercises to be part of your daily routine. This will insure that you incorporate better eyesight into your lifestyle rather than setting up a separate exercise routine that can easily become boring and a chore to do.

2. Start with simple fun things and small challenges to build confidence. Try eating or dressing without glasses. These things you can almost do with your eyes closed.

3. Whether you are nearsighted or farsighted, determine where the blur zone begins and challenge yourself to keep pushing that limit a little further. This might mean trying to play a game of cards or sitting just a little farther away from your TV.

4. Liken eye fitness to other fitness programs such as jogging or weight training. To condition yourself to run a mile, you have to work up to being able to complete the entire mile. It requires being attentive to the task and persistent. You will find that once you begin to rely less on glasses, your eyes will begin to accommodate and will get stronger. The old adage *use it or lose it* does apply to your eyes.

5. Use the eye exercises as additional flexibility challenges.

6. Keep a log or journal concerning your victories and your frustrations.

7. Remember that seeing clearly is part of balancing close work with more relaxed far focusing. Take breaks from close work and refocus.

8. Incorporate your eye training with sports or hobbies and recreation. Choose something that gives you visual practice. Ping pong, soccer, tennis, bicycling, kayaking, spectator sports or going to the movies can be part of your exercise. If you ride an exercise bike, use the time to focus on the wall chart across the room or try to see yourself clearly in the wall mirror.

9. Looking at the eye chart everyday is important in monitoring clarity of vision. Check your vision each morning with an eye chart to give you a reference point of how well you are seeing compared to yesterday, last week, or six months ago.

10. The real work comes when you are experimenting with your vision. What makes it clearer and what makes it less clear. Better sight is not necessarily effort but relaxing and paying attention to how clearly you are seeing. As you develop sensitivity for bringing something slightly out of focus into focus, you will develop the skills you need to see better.

Goals

Just as other fitness programs have different levels of achievement so does eye training. The runner may be content to run one mile, three times a week or may want to run in competition. Beginning levels of achievement may come about more quickly and easily than the final push for perfectly clear sight. So even if you have a strong prescription and are skeptical that vision training could help you, you may actually find that just by removing your glasses, your vision automatically improves. As Dr. Liberman points out in *Take Off Your Glasses and See,* "No matter how *weak* your eyesight is, you are very likely wearing your prescription more than you really need to. Most people find that there are very few activities that really require the full prescription that eye doctors are trained to provide, because those prescriptions are based on our worst-case visual need. Do we really need the same prescription to drive in a rainstorm at night as we do to read a book outside on a sunny day? Absolutely not!"

Goals for eye training can vary:

- Stopping further deterioration
- Improving sight & lowering your
     prescription
- Wearing glasses only when driving
- Complete effortless sight

Setting goals can help motivate you and can improve your progress. As you start finding that you can do things without your glasses, you start realizing that you can take on greater challenges.

Exercises

The normal eye, which has good vision, will be relaxed seeing both far and near with no strain. This means that the shape of the eye is round, eye muscles are flexible, strong, and well coordinated enough to accommodate for clear vision.

Relaxation Exercises:

Relaxation exercises give you an awareness of releasing tension. When eyesight is not clear, the eyes are not able to be as relaxed and seeing is more of a strain. Think about relaxation not as rest but as reducing strain. Even in sleep, our eyes are not necessarily relaxed because dream patterns keep our eyes in movement. I would like to draw an analogy of building vision fitness as a similar exercise to strength training. The weight lifter who builds his muscles gradually, so that he is actually relaxing into a lift rather than straining or jerking, is in control at all times and can easily do an exercise without injury.

Accommodation & Coordination Exercises:

As with any other fitness program, you have to push your level of fitness or flexibility by daily being aware of how clear or unclear things appear. In myopia, you tend to overfocus and you need to learn to relax the ciliary muscle and perhaps use the recti to pull the cornea flatter. In farsightedness you are underfocusing and need to relax the recti, which flatten the cornea too much, and develop coordination of the oblique and ciliary muscles. Both near and far vision can show improvement by doing the exercises and paying attention to how clearly you are seeing.

Balance:

The third part is balancing your activities to give your eyes a chance to use all of their powers everyday. This will not only help your eyesight but will insure a more balanced lifestyle.

Chinese posters in factories and schools recommend massaging at acupuncture points as defined in Chinese medicine to stimulate circulation.

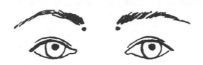

Massage under bone ridge at inside corners of the eyebrow using fingers.

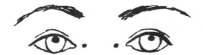

Massage bridge of nose using index fingers.

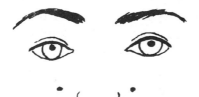

Place index fingers on cheek bones approximately one finger distance from the nose and massage gently.

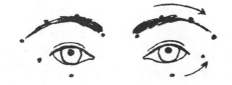

Massage outward along brow bone and under eye along bone ridge to outer corner of eye with fingers.

Relaxation Exercises

Bates included these types of exercises in his books. The objective of these exercises is to reduce strain and tension in the eyes and body.

Covering Eyes with Palms

Rub the hands together to warm the palms. Close your eyes and place the palms over the eyes. The hands should rest lightly on the bony ridges around the eyes, but should not touch the eyelids.

Relax in the Sun

Find a comfortable place to sit in the sun. Close the eyes and feel the light warm the eyelids. Allow yourself to relax and enjoy the experience. If you like, you can also move your head from side to side to relax the neck muscles.

Relaxed Movement

Stand with feet slightly apart. Rhythmically rotate the body, twisting so that your head and shoulders are looking from side to side. Let your arms swing in a relaxed manner at your sides and keep your eyes open so that the world appears to be spinning past your gaze. Allow your whole body to relax.

Look out a Window

I did not find palming worked very well. Instead I find that my eyes relax instantly if I go over to the window and look out into the brighter full spectrum natural light. When I return to the chart in the hall I can keep the relaxation going and the letters on the chart clear.

Why Relaxation Works

Muscle tension associated with close work usually plays a part in why people begin wearing corrective lenses for nearsightedness, farsightedness, and astigmatism. By learning to let go and release the tension, you free up the eyes to be flexible so they can more easily respond to automatic focusing reflexes.

Stereograms have recently become popular. These are two dimensional pictures which strangely appear three dimensional when you relax your focus. See if you can see the hidden 3-D picture in the stereogram on the next page.

To see this hidden image, focus your eyes on something across the room. Without losing that focus point, bring the stereogram in front of your face. Slowly move it away from your eyes. The image may be a little blurry at first, but your eyes should gradually find the stereogram's focus point.

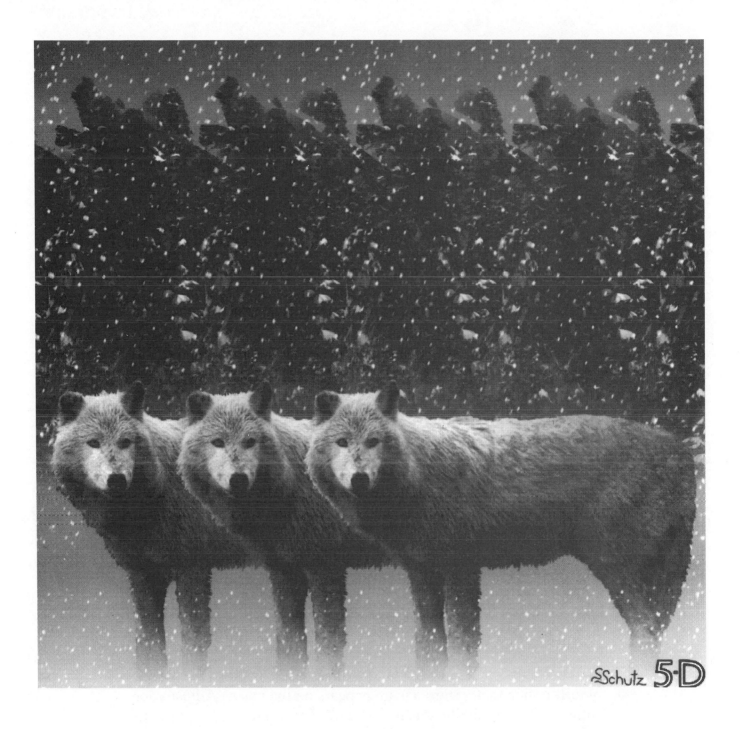

Hi Squares - (Myopia, Hyperopia, Astigmatism, & Presbyopia)

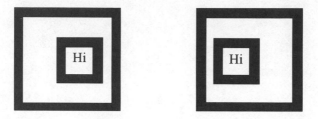

A similar exercise was recommended in both Dr. Hutchinson's book, *Computer Eye Stress, How to Avoid It, How to Alleviate It*, and in Dr. Kaplan's book, *Seeing Beyond 20/20*. I don't know where it actually originated.

This exercise is an effective exercise for both farsighted and nearsighted problems. There is a connection between the crossing muscles and the focusing muscles. If you are farsighted, you are underfocusing and, if you are nearsighted, you are overfocusing. This exercise helps your coordination.

Instructions:
Hold the squares a comfortable distance from your eyes. Cross your eyes slightly so that three squares appear on the page. Adjust your vision until you can read the word "Hi" clearly in the center. Notice that the center appears to recede.

Once you master the eye-crossing phase, you can try doing the exercise using your far vision. This time look into the distance and bring the squares up between your eyes and the distant object of your focus. Keep your attention focused far away. Again, you'll notice that a third square appears on the page. Adjust your sight until the middle square is clear. The center may appear to advance.

If you have mastered the exercises above, try doing them again, but this time try moving the page toward you and away from you while keeping the middle square in focus.

Variant on Hi Squares - (Myopia)

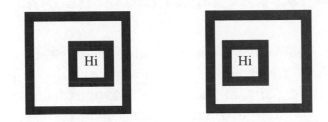

This exercise is a variant of the HI SQUARES exercise, however, I have modified it slightly so that it became more effective for me while working with myopia. This exercise helps train the eyes to use the crossing and focusing muscles together for distance.

Instructions:
First learn how to comfortably do the HI SQUARES exercise so that you can create the third square both while crossing your eyes and using your far vision. You must also be able to hold the visual image while moving the paper closer and further from you. If you can, you are ready to expand the exercise by increasing the distance.

Tape this exercise on the wall next to the eye chart. Now perform the exercises while stepping back from the chart and hold the image. You should do both crossed and far-focus. You can pick up the far-focus by touching your nose on the page between the HI SQUARES and step back. Learn to blink while still holding the image so that you can let your eyes break when needed. It is possible to step back twenty feet while still holding the image. As you train your eyes to work together moving farther and farther from the wall, you may begin to see that after doing this exercise the eye chart is much clearer. (If I have been doing close work and find my sight blurry, I can immediately improve my far focus by doing this exercise.)

Concentric Circles Exercise - (Astigmatism)

This exercise helps you see your whole field of vision at once, which makes you aware of how you are distorting parts of the image. Astigmatism affects how you see horizontal or vertical lines. Working with the image to bring it all into clear focus increases your flexibility. At first, it may appear that the breaks in the circle are immobile but, by simply relaxing your gaze, you may notice the image change.

If you have astigmatism, you will notice that the bull's eye becomes distorted at a distance. It may have lines through it and begin to look like a kaleidoscope at a distance instead of appearing as a series of increasingly larger continuous bands of alternating color.

Stand where you can comfortably see the center clearly and notice that the concentric circles continue all around the circle. Now move back to where the circles begin to break. Try to relax and adjust your focus to bring the center of the chart into clear view. Keep moving into the blur zone and bring the chart back into focus. Another thing you can try is focusing on a band near the outer edge of the circle. Move your eyes around the circle, trying to see the continuous colored band continuing through the breaks. It may seem impossible to move through the breaks at first but, once you do, you will find that your vision becomes far more flexible. Soon you will soon be able to clear the circle easily.

Post this exercise next to your eye chart so you can look back and forth between the two as you work. This way you can check the clarity on both charts.

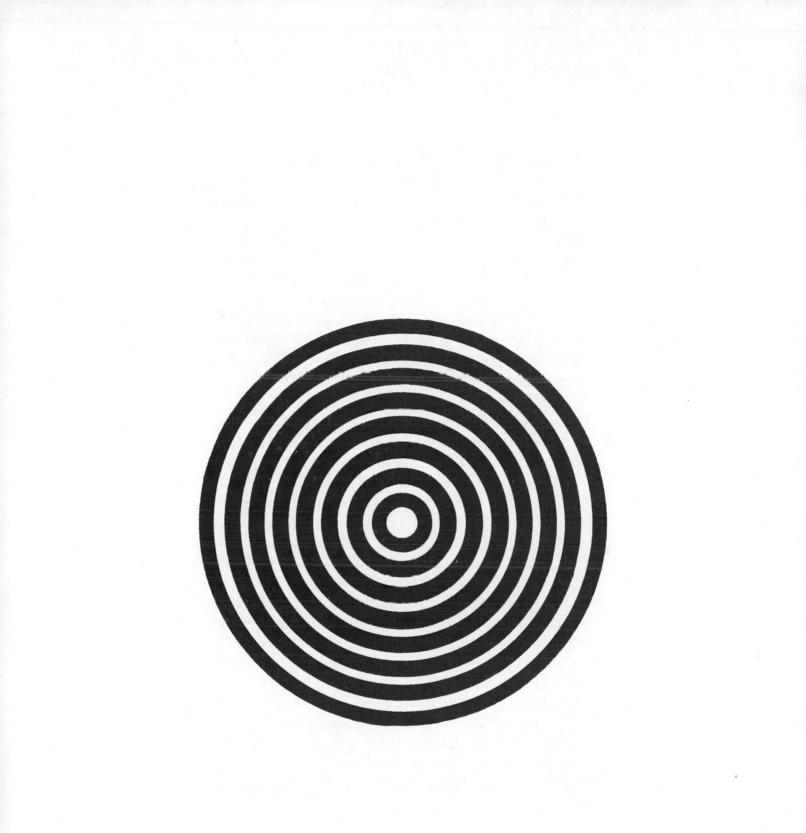

Diagonal Lines Exercise - (Astigmatism)

One day I noticed that I had trouble seeing diagonals. If a sign contained the letters "V, N, S, M, etc.," at a distance the diagonal lines would bunch together and fade out, and I consequently had a hard time reading them. This eye exercise is similar to the bull's eye exercise and helps you see how your vision may be distorted. The objective of this exercise is to help you practice adjusting your sight so that the white and black lines appear equally uniform in size and are sharp and clear.

Practice with each eye separately, then both together. Stand where you can see the diagonal chart clearly. Then move back and see if the chart starts to distort. Can you continue to see the white lines (nice and fat) as if they were threads running through a woven piece of burlap? Can you see the diamond shapes black and clear in the background?

An eye doctor once told me that my eyes tended to look inward slightly (toward my nose). I found that when I practiced, one eye at a time, looking at the chart by moving my focus more toward the corner of my eye, the diagonal lines became less distorted. After practicing with the chart for a week, my coordination dramatically improved. I no longer had to exaggerate the movement; I began to focus on the diagonals easily. Use this chart to train your eyes to see the images clearly without distortion. This exercise might help you clear up the blur zones in the bull's eye.

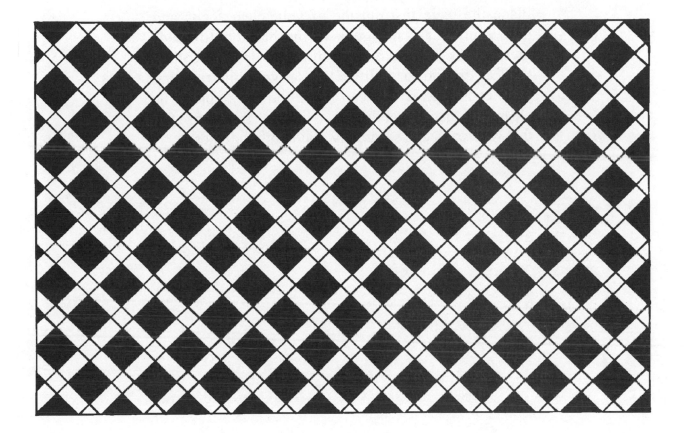

Black Lines - (Nearsightedness & Astigmatism)

Place the page just outside of your clear focus and into your blur zone. Look at the black outlines of these forms. If parts of the outline are unclear, follow the line around that part of the design while relaxing your eyes. See if you can make the lines appear as clear and distinct as the other lines of the form. Try this with each eye separately, then both together.

The Wave - (Nearsightedness & Astigmatism)

Place the page somewhere in your blur zone. Look at the page and see if you can see the uniform wave pattern running across the page. Both white and black lines should look the same width and be continuous. You may want to move more or less into the blur zone. Work at seeing the waves clearly with each eye. Try to make the contrast of black and white sharper. Now turn the page sideways so that the lines run up and down. Check to see if it is easier to see the waves in this position.

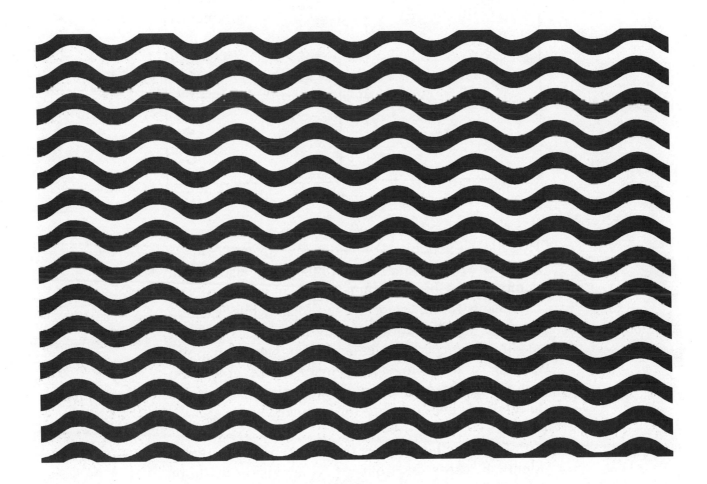

Cards - (Myopia)

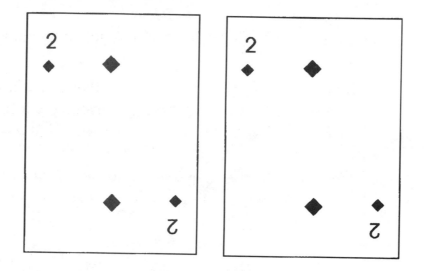

A similar exercise is recommended in Dr. Hutchinson's book, *Computer Eye Stress, How to Avoid It, How to Alleviate It*, but I have also seen it demonstrated by Dr. Kaplan. The objective of this exercise is to train your eyes to focus while learning to move the eyes outward away from your nose. For reading, the eye muscles are strenghtened to point inward to focus together. This exercise gives you practice coordinating and strengthening the muscles to focus the eyes outward for distance vision.

Look at something across the room and hold up two identical cards in front of your vision without changing your focus. Notice that a third card appears in between the original two. Bring the third card into focus so that it is identical to the original two images. Try to hold the third card in focus as you move the cards first closer to you and then away from you. Now, see how long you can hold the image of the third card as you begin widening the distance between the two cards.

Fine Print - (Hyperopia & Presbyopia)

The objective of this exercise is to practice focusing on print.

Start by working with a type size that you can read without glasses. Look at the white space inside the letter and try to make it whiter and clearer by relaxing your eyes.

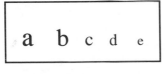

Trace around the border of the box, then go back to the letter and try to bring it into clearer focus.

Move to a smaller letter or bring the page closer so the type slightly blurs. Try to bring the slightly blurry print into clearer focus. Look back at a larger letter.

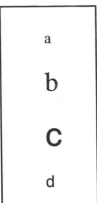

Cover one eye with a card, or your hand, to work on one eye at a time. When you lose focus, relax your eyes by looking at something across the room and then refocus on the print. You can also relax by moving your eyes along the white space around the letters.

z	y	x	w	v
F	U	N	n	y
k	l	m	n	o
p	q	r	s	t
A	E	I	O	U

Remember to take breaks from reading and look up often to refocus. Long periods of close work cause near point stress for all eyes.

Patterns – (Farsightedness)

Try bringing these patterns into focus with each eye separately, then both together. Start with the designs at a comfortable distance, then move them closer to make it more difficult. If you lose the focus, move the paper farther away and start again. You can find your own interesting designs to work with or try an amusing cartoon.

$ j I {>? rc @ ^ ! ~ % +

*** /// ||| \\\ ***

Additional Available Aids

Biofeedback Training

In the 1980s, Dr. Joseph Trachtman invented and patented the Accommotrac vision training devise to help cure myopia. It is a biofeedback machine that makes a noise to inform a person when the ciliary muscle relaxes, which can in turn improve distance sight. The Accommotrac is available through many vision therapists around the country. The training has proved effective and is now being used to cure many other visual problems in addition to myopia; however, it is more expensive than the books and other methods that I have included herein.

Lenses as Resistance Training

Brian Severson, an engineer and pilot, recently devised a method using lenses as a resistance force (like weights) to strengthen the eyesight. Brian's dream was to become an airline pilot. In order to be competitive in his desire to work for a major airline, he needed to obtain a college degree. Unfortunately, the amount of reading required to get his engineering degree worked against him. Although he practiced good vision habits, he became nearsighted and was unable to pass the 20/20 vision test, which was a requirement at the time. Brian did not give up. After years of research, he developed a technique using reading glasses as resistance to strengthen his distance sight. He became a pilot for United Airlines, but markets his course to help others achieve better vision.

I have used his *Vision Freedom* method and found it very helpful in correcting my sight. He originally was working on a cure for his own myopia, but has found the same principles apply to other visual problems. I would recommend this method as an additional option in your quest to become less dependent on glasses. Brian has a patent pending and sells a reasonably priced kit that includes a book describing his techniques. I have included his address and phone number in the bibliography at the back of this book.

Behavioral Optometrists

Several of the books listed in the bibliography were written by behavioral optometrists. Their roots go back to the turn of the century. They have carried on the tradition of vision improvement through the use of education about lifestyle, nutrition, proper use of glasses, and practice of visual exercises and psychologically based drills. They may be able to assist you with vision correction techniques and a slightly weaker prescription so your eyes will be able to practice adjusting for the difference. Approximately one-eighth of practicing optometrists in the U.S. are behavioral optometrists.

Student Observations & Suggestions

I developed this book as a learning tool to use in a six hour course I taught for the past year in an evening community education program. I've learned a lot from the participants' comments about their experiences. Here are some of their observations.

One night a male college student mentioned that his studies forced him to stare at equations when he was working on mathematical problems. He wondered if there was anything he could do about this. Another student in the class suggested that he get a black board or a magic marker board so that he could write out the equations in large print. Then he could sit across the room while he pondered the solutions.

A woman found that her distance sight improved when she returned to college after working for a few years. She felt that the daily time she spent in class looking at the board or viewing an overhead projection was making the difference. This practice of far focusing was giving her the varied visual movement that she did not experience in her job.

Before attending my class, one young woman had been practicing relaxation techniques, but found her progress had stalled. She especially liked the *Concentric Circles* and the *Diagonal Lines Exercises* since they gave her some specific visual feedback and offered her a new way to address her distorted vision.

One college student decided to take my advise and walk around campus while resting his eyes. He said that after he finishes studying, his distance sight is sometimes noticeably blurrier than normal, but after a short while his normal acuity usually returns. He was hoping to learn how to retain his good eyesight. He's taken a big step by becoming aware of how he sees and what affects his ability to see.

During the first session of my classes, I usually have the students describe why they chose to take the class as a way for the students to get to know each other. One woman mentioned that she had been wearing glasses since grade school for nearsightedness. She said she wore her glasses all the time. When I suggested that she try to read without wearing her glasses, she expressed concern about getting headaches. I encouraged her to just try it for a few minutes. Two weeks later the woman mentioned that she was elated at the change. She had been reading without her glasses; since she had been monitoring her distance sight with a chart, she was amazed that she saw a noticeable improvement in her distance vision. She hoped that she could continue this. Since your eyes have to accommodate over your distance prescription to read, you tend to strengthen your eyes in the wrong direction if you wear them for close work. By taking your glasses off and moving the book farther away, you start emulating the habits of a farsighted person. This is the same concept that the Vision Freedom method employes.

I noticed also that when I stopped wearing my contacts, which corrected for distance, even my computer screen was blurry. Since I was already experimenting with my distance acuity, I decided to see if my eyes would accommodate to this near point blur as well. Within a week, my eyes had already accommodated to clear up the computer screen. Now I still practice this concept and work with my computer screen farther away.

When I started to improve my distance vision I noted

that the eye chart was blurry at twelve feet, but also that type on my computer was blurry. Everything in between was blurry to some degree. After a while, I recognized that I didn't have to be twenty feet away from a chart to work on my distance vision. I could work on small type at arms length and my TV screen at ten feet or anything in between that was noticeably distorted. Letters or geometric lines and curves are good to work with since they give you a good indication of visual clarity.

Bibliography

Bates, William. *The Bates Method for Better Eyesight Without Glasses*. New York: Holt, Rinehart, & Winston, 1981.

Corbett, Margaret Darst. *Help Yourself to Better Sight*. North Hollywood, CA: Wilshire Book Co., 1949.

Godnig, Edward & John Hacunda. *Computers and Visual Stress*. Seacoast Information Services, Inc., Charlestown, Rhode Island, 1990.

Goodrich, Janet. *NaturalVision Improvement*. Berkeley, CA: Celestial Arts, 1985.

Hutchinson, R. Anthony. *Computer Eye Stress, How to Avoid It, How to Alleviate It*. New York: M. Evans, 1985.

Huxley, Aldous. *The Art of Seeing*. Berkeley, CA: Creative Arts Book Company, 1982 .

Kaplan, Robert-Michael. *Seeing Beyond 20/20*. Hillsboro, OR: Beyond Words Publishing, Inc., 1987.

Leviton, Richard. *Seven Stops to Better Vision*. Brookline, Mass: East West / Natural Health Books, 1992.

Liberman, Jacob. *Take Off Your Glasses & See*. New York: Crown Publishing, Inc., 1995.

Mansfield, Peter. *The Bates Method*. United Kingdom: Optima, 1995

Rosanes-Berrett, Marilyn. *Do You Really Need Eyeglasses?* New York: I.I., Inc., 1983

Seiderman, Arthur & Steven Marcus. *20/20 Is Not Enough.* New York: Fawcett Crest/Ballantine Books, 1989

Severson, Brian. *Vision Freedom*. 1665 Red Crow Road, Victor, Montana 59875, 1994. 406-961-5570.

For additional copies of *EyeRobics*
please send $14.95 plus shipping & handling,
and sales tax if applicable to:

EYESercise
P.O. Box 9544
Seattle WA 98109
or online - www.eyesercise.com

Ship to: Name_____ Telephone # _____

Street_____

City_____State_____Zip_____

Quantity_____of books @ $14.95 each = _____

(Washington Residents Add 8.2%) Sales Tax = _____

($3.50 for one copy, plus $1.50 for each   Shipping & Handling = _____
additional copy sent to the same address.)

Total = _____

I will pay by:

☐ Visa   ☐ Enclosed Check
☐ MasterCard   ☐ Enclosed Money Order

(Make check or money order payable to EyeRobics)

Credit Card No.   __ __ __ __ __ __ __ __ __ __ __ __ __ __ __ __

Expiration Date:_____Card Holder's Signature_____

Please list additional copies to be sent to other
addresses on a separate sheet.